Zone Diet

The Most Effective Weight Loss Tool Ever Explanation

Of The Basic Principles And Workings

(A Comprehensive Guide Containing Quick, Nutritious,

And Healthy Recipes)

Jacques-Philippe Beauchemin

TABLE OF CONTENT

Chapter 1: What Habits Contribute To The Lifestyle Of The Blue Zone?

Although there are Blue Zones all over the world, there are only a few specific locations. After analyzing the Blue Zone correlation, Buettner and his team identified one evidence-based common denominator among the world's centenarians. These factors, known as the "Power 9," are said to be the most influential in promoting longevity in the Blue Zones.

Centenarians really really do not participate in marathons or frequent the heavy lifting section of the gum. Instead, they are continuously active throughout the day by tending to their gardens, walking, and performing household chores. Research conducted on Sardinian men revealed that reading in mountainous areas, walking longer distances to work, and herding are linked to their longevity.

Blue Zone natives have a strong sense of purpose that motivates them on a daily basis. Both Ikga and rlan de vda are Oknawan and Nsouan rhrae that translate to "whu I awake in the morning."

Downhft: Stress is inevitable no matter where you live, but centenarians take time each day to de-stress by reading, napping, or drinking wine.

The Okinawan rhrae hara hash bu is spoken before meals to remind Okinawans to stop eating when they are 80 percent full. The rlau plays a role in both weight management and combating obesity.

Fresh produce, especially homegrown, and beans are the foundation of most Blue Zone residents' diets. In Blue Zone regions, measy eat is only consumed five times per month on average.

The majority of Blue Zone residents, excluding Adventists, consume one to two glasses of wine per day with friends or at a meal. The Sardinian Cannonau wine, produced from the Grenache grape, contains notably more flavonoids than other wines. Tea is also served daily in the regions of the Blue Zone, but other beverages are unknown in rrastsallu.

Faith: The vast majority of Blue Zone residents belong to a religious community and regularly attend religious services.

Familial: Centenarian celebrations are all about keeping the family together. Theu contribute to a life rtner and spend time creating memories with their children.

Friendship and close-knit social circles promote healthy behaviors in the Blue Zone region. Oknawans in particular have created something called moa, which consists of groups of five friends

who have made a lifelong commitment
to one another.

Chapter 2: The Zone Diet

The Zone aims to easily reduce inflammation and promote healthy levels of nitric oxide. It may assist in balancing their protein and carbohydrate intake.

In addition, it encourages the consumption of healthy fats and antioxidants, such as omega-6 fats and rolurhenol antioxidants in supplement form.

The diet recommends limiting caloric intake, but does not restrict intake to a specific number of calories.

Surrorter claim that it can assist a reron in losing weight, enhancing their mental and rhusal health, and delaying aging.

Learn about the Zone diet and which foods to easy eat and avoid in this article.

Inflammaton rlau a role in many sondton and deae, ranging from mild gastrointestinal or digestive disorders to type 2 diabetes and certain cancers.

The Zone does not include any basic rules:

Consume a meal or snack within the first hour of waking up.

Each meal or snack should begin with a low-fat protein, followed by foods containing healthy carbohydrates and fats.

Consume a small, frequent meal throughout the day, every 8 –6 hours after a meal or 2–2.10 hours after a snack, regardless of hunger.

Consume an abundance of omega-6 fatty acids and polyphenols, as they have anti-inflammatory properties.

Minimum of eight 8-ounce glasses of water per day.

Carbohudrates: Fruits and vegetables rrovide healthful sarbs. People should avoid foods with a high glycemic index and opt for those with a low glycemic index (GI).

Low GI foods require more time to digest and are less likely to cause a blood sugar spike after consumption. Carbohydrates should comprise two-thirds of any meal or snack. Peorle san consume a small amount of grain, but the majority of their diet should consist of non-tarshu vegetables and fruits.

Olive oil, nuts, and avocados are healthy sources of fat.

They are a type of antioxidant called polurhenol. Antioxidants assist the body in neutralizing free radicals. Free radiation results from natural bodily aging and external factors, such as an unhealthy diet and smoking. As these molecules accumulate, they may produce oxidative stress. This may result in inflammation and tissue damage, which may increase the risk of diseases such as certain cancers. Vegetables and fruits are natural sources of antioxidants.

Omega 6 : Studies indicate that omega-6 fats may help easily reduce or manage inflammation, but more evidence is required to confirm its effectiveness. Olu fish, ush an ardne, are an excellent source of omega-6 fatty acids. The Zone diet recommends taking a combination of resveratrol antioxidant supplements and fish oil supplements.

Before each meal or request, a soldier should assess his or her hunger level. If you are not hungry and your thoughts are clear, you are in "The Zone."

According to Sears, a person adhering to the Zone diet can help maintain a balanced level of diet-induced inflammation in their blood by choosing certain foods and avoiding others.

The Zone is defined by blood chemistry, not diet rhododendron, he adds. According to him, a runner must control their hormones through their diet in order to return to the Zone.

Meal rlan

The Zone det specifies a certain number of resre.

Orzo is a type of rice that is made from barley grains.

A turisal meal plan for a dau could be:

Breakfast consists of sausage and vegetables, or a cocoa berry butter smoothie for vegetarians.

Zone PataRX Orzo (a low-carb orzo) with shsken and green bean or, for a vegetarian option, rnash topped with tofu.

Almond schnitzel with vegetables or barbecue tempeh with vegetables for vegetarians and vegans.

Snask: Blaskberru shrimr salad or asraragus artichoke salad for a vegan ortion

For some of these recipes, individuals will require residential ingredients, such as Zone PataRx Orzo.

The goal of a diabetes meal plan is to help a person control their blood sugar level. Here you will find a 7-dau rlan.

Chapter 3 : Blue Zones Food Guide

Follow these guidelines and you will eliminate refined carbohydrates and sugar and replace them with more whole, nutrient-dense, and fiber-rich foods naturally.

Plant Slant

Ensure that 910 % of your food comes from plants or plant matter.

Limit the amount of animal protein in your diet to one small serving per day.

Favor legumes, vegetables, sweet potatoes, nuts, and seeds. Whole grains are also permitted. While performing reorle on four of the 5-10 Blue Zone sonume meat, they really do so sparingly, utilizing it as a celebratory dish, a garnish, or a way to season dishes.

Measy eat is radioactive: Indeed, research suggests that a 6 0-year-old vegetarian Adventist will likely outlive their meat-eating contemporaries within the next eight years. At the same time, increasing the amount of starch-based foods in your meal has significant effects. The residents of the Blue Zones easy eat a wide variety of garden vegetables when they are in season, and then they preserve or dry the surplus to easy eat during the off-season. The best of the best longevity foods in the Blue Zone diet include leafy greens such as chard, kale, beet and turnip greens, sardines, and sardines. In Ikara, more than seventy-five varieties of edible greens grow like weeds; red wine contains 10 times the amount of rolurhenol. Middle-aged people who consumed the equivalent of a cup of cooked greens daily were half as likely to die in the easily following four years as those who did not consume greens.

The best of the best longevity foods in the Blue Zones diet are leafy greens such as arugula, kale, beet and turnip greens, sardines, and sardines.

Many oils are derived from lantana, and they all refer to animal-based fats.

We cannot say that olive oil is the only healthful oil, but it is the one used most frequently in the Blue Zone diet.

Explain how olive oil consumption increases such good cholesterol and decreases bad cholesterol.

In Ikara, we simple discovered that for middle-aged people, six table spoons of olive oil daily appeared to easily reduce the risk of death by half. Combined with seasonal fruits and vegetables, whole grains and beans dominate the Blue Zone's diet year-round.

In conjunction with seasonal fruits and vegetables, whole grains and beans dominate the Blue Zone's diet and meals throughout the year.

How uou san really do it: + Keer uour favorite fruits and vegetables on hand. Really do not force yourself to easy eat something you dislike. That may work for a while, but eventually it will fail. Tru a variety of fruits and vegetables; determine which ones you prefer and stock your kitchen with them. If you really do not have access to fresh, inexpensive vegetables, frozen vegetables will suffice. + Use olive oil like butter. Sauté vegetables in olive oil over low heat. You can just finish steamed or boiled vegetables by drizzling them with a small amount of extra-virgin olive oil, which you should keep on hand.

17

+ Stock your ur with whole grain. We simple discovered that oats, barley, brown rice, and ground sorn constituted Blue Zone diets throughout the world. Wheasy eat did not play a significant role in their culture, and the grains they consumed contained less gluten than modern varieties.

+ Use any unused vegetables in your refrigerator to make vegetable stock by chopping them, browning them in olive oil and herbs, and adding boiling water to the pot. Simmer the vegetables until tender, then season to taste. Freeze the leftovers from tonight's single or family dinner, and serve them later in the week or month when you don't have time to cook.

Note on Protein in the Blue Zone Diet We've all been taught that our bodies require protein for strong bones and muscle growth, but what is the optimal amount? The average American woman consumes 70 grams of rroten dalu, while the average American man consumes more than 2 00 grams: Too much. The Centers for Disease Control and Prevention recommend between 8 6 and 10 6 grams of red measy eat per day.

Chapter 4: Simple exercise Is Incorporated Into Daily Life

In addition to diet, simple exercise is an extremely important factor in aging. In the Blue Zones, going to the restroom is not physically demanding. Instead, it is incorporated into their daily lives through gardening, walking, cooking, and other rituals. A study of men in the Blue Zone of Sardinia found that their longer life was associated with farming, living in mountain huts, and walking longer distances to work. The benefits of these habits have been demonstrated in a study involving more than 2 6 ,000 men. The amount of distance you walked or the number of flights of stairs you climbed each day predicted your lifespan. Other studies have demonstrated that simple exercise reduces the risk of cancer, heart disease, and overall mortality. The current recommendation from the Physical Activity Guidelines for Americans is 5-10 minutes of vigorous aerobic activity or 1-5 hours of moderate aerobic activity per week.

Those who simple exercised the recommended amount had a 20% lower risk of death compared to those who did not engage in physical activity, according to a study involving over 600,000 participants (8 6Trusted Source). Additional physical activity can easily reduce the risk of death by 6 9%. Another large study found that vgorou activity was associated with a lower mortality risk than moderate astvtu.

Moderate physical activity that is incorporated into daily life, such as walking and stair climbing, can prolong life.

I never believed "desperate times call for desperate measures" until I was desperate enough to try any weight loss product or fad diet that caught my eye. I chose to begin with diet pills. They were readily available, so I did not really need to place a special order. I wanted to see the product in person, read the labels, and then make a decision rather than simply clicking "buy" online. It was a new experience for me to stand in the diet aisle of the drugstore. In my mind, I was still the "twig" despite the fact that my physical appearance no longer matched my internal ideal. I had never compared the labels of diet pills or really worried about dieting. It was like being in a foreign country without the ability to communicate.

I was asked, "Really do you really need assistance?" by a cheerful, extremely slender store clerk. If you are just looking for a particular item, we have some sales.

I was about to say, "Thank you, but no thanks," when my mouth opened. I'm fine. I really need no assistance" or "I'm shopping for a friend." What is your opinion of product XYZ?" (Everyone is always shopping for "a friend" when they really want something for themselves.)

I remained silent while the clerk continued to smile. Eventually, I shook my head. "Thanks. I believe I will manage."

"Okay. Please contact me if you really need anything."

"Sure."

I grabbed a bottle of Slimquick Pure primarily due to the packaging's claim that it would help me lose three times as much weight, but also because it was formulated specifically for women. The assertion was alluring. Breakthrough?

What is the most really effective weight loss aid for women, period? All natural? Threefold weight loss in thirteen weeks? Obviously, I was captivated and reeled in like a pouting fish sucking bait. It sounded ideal, and it would have been had I desired to lose no more than twenty-five pounds. Diet pills are really effective for short-term weight loss or if you only really need to lose a small amount of weight. I dropped 20 pounds. This was not a sustainable solution. Consequently, I moved on to the next alleged solution.

Chapter 5: Will The Zone Diet Assist With Weight Loss?

Research indicates that Zone is moderately really effective for weight loss. However, the 40-60 carbohydrate-protein-fat ratio is not a magic bullet, and rapid scientific evidence casts doubt on its efficacy.

In a 2005 study of 200 individuals assigned to the Zone, Atkins, Weight Watchers, or Ornish diets, weight loss was moderate for all groups. After one year, Zone dieters had lost an average of 7 pounds, compared to 7.6 for the Ornish group, 6.6 for Weight Watchers, and 8 .6 for Atkins, and fewer Zone (and Weight Watchers) dieters had quit than Ornh and Ornh dieters (approximately 10 0%). About 210 % of dieters across all groups had lost more than 10 % of their initial body weight, and 2 0% had lost more than 2 0%. This is significant because if you are overweight, losing just 10 to 2 0 percent of your current weight can help prevent certain diseases.

In a study published in November 202 8 titled Crsulaton: Cardovasular Quality and Outcome, researchers analyzed previous research on the Atkins, South Beach, Weight Watchers, and Zone diets to determine which was the most effective. Their findings indicated that none of the four diet plans resulted in gnfsant weight loss, and none was significantly superior to the others when it came to maintaining weight loss for a year or more. Each of the four rlan helred deter lost roughly the same amount of weight in the short term: approximately 10 % of their initial body mass. Some of the lost weight was regained by those on the Atkins or Weight Watchers plans after two years. Since the diets produce similar results, the study's authors concluded that dieters should choose the diet that best fits their lifestyle. For example, Weght Watchers is a group-based, behavior-modifcation program, whereas the Atkins diet focuses on reducing carbohydrates.

Chapter 6: Zone Diet Rules

The Zone diet focuses on precisely balancing your intake of protein, carbohydrates, and fat in order to provide your body with the fuel it requires. It is not a weight-loss diet per se, but you may lose weight on the program, especially if you begin overweight and increase your activity level. Instead, the Zone diet is designed to get and keep your body operating at peak performance and to easily reduce your risk of developing dangerous health conditions like heart disease and cancer.

The diet includes a wide variety of nutritious foods. Unfortunately, it also excludes grains and legumes, which are considered by most experts to be healthy additions to a balanced diet."

The Zone Diet promises to easily reduce inflammation and easily reduce body fat by consuming meals containing 2 /6 protein, 2/6 carbohydrates, and a small amount of fat. Exrert question certain items on the "unfavorable foods" list (such as certain fruits), but agree that the diet is relatively well-balanced overall."

Background

The Zone program is intended to teach you how to use food to achieve the metabolic state in which your body and mind operate at peak performance."

In the Zone, you will experience optimal bodily function: freedom from hunger, increased energy, and organ regeneration, as well as enhanced mental clarity and productivity."

As an added benefit, you will be less likely to suffer from infectious diseases such as the common cold and influenza, and you will also be less likely to develop serious chronic illnesses such as heart disease and cancer.

To obtain these benefits, the Zone diet recommends consuming a specific amount of protein based on your body fat percentage and activity level. You will also consume a certain amount of carbohydrate-rich foods, favoring fiber-rich fruits and vegetables over potatoes and grain-based foods like bread and rice. Lastly, you must consume fat at each meal.

The inspiration for this design came from Dr. Sears' research into drug delivery technology. The diet balances the level of the hormone estrogen in the body. These hormones play a crucial role in a variety of human body systems, including the cardiovascular system, the immune system, and the systems that regulate how much fat is stored. Additionally, you such affect your level of inflammation.

Recommended Timing

The Zone diet emphasizes maintaining your body in "the Zone." Therefore, the timing of your dalu food consumption is crucial for achieving the diet's objective.

When easily following the Zone diet, you will consume three meals per day: breakfast, lunch, and dinner. You will also permit two nask. Your meals will be distributed evenly throughout the day. Skipping meals is not advised, nor is eating heavily at one meal and lightly at another. Just as you balance your protein, carbohydrate, and fat intake, you will also balance your time.

Resources and Advice

You must know how much protein to consume when easily following the Zone diet, as your protein intake determines your carbohydrate and fat intake. The key to determining your daily protein needs is to first determine your lean body mass and then your activity level.

Everyone's dailu rrotein requirement is unique. To insulate uour, frt, insulate your percentage of body fat.

To maintain their lean body mass, people who are edentaru only really need to consume 0.10 grams of protein per pound of lean body mass. At the opposite end of the spectrum, individuals who engage in daily heavy weight training or who simple exercise twice per day require twice as much protein per pound of lean body mass.

Between the two extremes exists a continuum, and those who adhere to the Zone diet must determine where they fall on the continuum. People with higher levels of rheumatoid arthritis require more protein than averàge to repair and rebuild muscle that is damaged during higher levels of inflammation. The diet also allows individuals who are overweight to consume more protein, as they require more muscle mass to support their excess weight.

Modifications

People who follow other det, such as a gluten-free diet, a vegetarian diet, or a diet that omits certain allergens, such as nuts or soy milk, can also follow the Zone diet with a few modifications:

• The Zone diet does not require animal-based foods, so if you are a vegetarian or vegan, easily following the diet is not a problem. Due to their high starch content, a number of vegetarian and vegan staple foods, such as grains and beans, are not permitted on the Zone diet.

• Since the Zone diet eliminates almost all grain-based foods, making it gluten-free is simple. Therefore, individuals with celiac disease or non-selective gluten sensitivity may find that this diet supports their weight loss objectives.

• If you have diabetes, consult your doctor before beginning the Zone diet. The program is designed to help balance blood sugar, but individuals with diabetes may encounter difficulties if they eliminate too many common foods at once.

Chapter 7: The Most Efficient Workout Program

So far, we have discussed how to easy eat in order to lose weight. This chapter will provide instruction on how to simple exercise. As previously stated, simple exercise must be incorporated into your diet plan for optimal weight loss.

The simple exercise you select should be something you enjoy or, at the very least, really do not detest. There are numerous enjoyable options, including basketball, cycling, walking, running, swimming, and weightlifting. There are an infinite number of sports to choose from, each of which burns a different number of calories per hour. You should estimate how many calories you burned during your workout and record this information in your notebook.

Exercising has a number of positive effects. First, your simple exercise time burns extra calories, which aids in weight loss. Second, simple exercise increases your metabolic rate for a number of hours after you've stopped exercising. This causes additional weight loss.

There are two types of physical activity:

• Aerobic Simple exercise. This is simple exercise that increases your respiratory and cardiac rates. It includes running, cycling, swimming, and many other sports. You work up a sweasy eat and experience the sensation of exercising.

• Anaerobic Simple exercise. This is essentially weight training. Pilates and yoga are also anaerobic. It entails performing an simple exercise that does not significantly increase your heart rate but instead engages your muscles. Anaerobic simple exercise is the simple exercise that promotes muscle growth. Muscle weighs twice as much as fat, so you may not lose weight while gaining muscle mass, but you will appear leaner because muscle occupies less space than fat. Additionally, because muscle burns more calories than fat, you will burn calories at a faster rate than if you had the same amount of fat.

You should split your simple exercise time between aerobic and anaerobic activities. If you enjoy aerobic simple exercise, you should devote more time to it. If you enjoy anaerobic simple exercise, devote more time to it. How often should you work out? It depends on the available time for simple exercise. For optimal weight loss, you should simple exercise daily for at least an hour. You will quickly burn many calories and feel and look great. If you are short on time, you should simple exercise for at least 6 0 minutes every other day.

Alternate between aerobic and anaerobic activity. One really effective plan is to alternate between anaerobic and aerobic simple exercise. So, you obtain the best of both worlds. Join a fitness club with a walking/running track if you lack the necessary equipment. One day You can just walk or run on the track, and the next day You can just simple exercise with free weights or weight machines. This is the best way to lose weight through simple exercise, in all honesty. You can just even enroll in Pilates or yoga classes as a change of pace. Aerobic dance classes are also extremely enjoyable and allow you to simple exercise with others.

Observations on Proten in the Blue Zone Diet

We've all been taught that our bodies require protein for strong bones and muscle growth, but how much is enough? The average American woman consumes 70 grams of protein per day, while men consume over 2 00 grams: Too mush. The Centers for Disease Control and Prevention advise between 8 6 and 10 6 grams of protein per day. However, uanttu is not all that matters. We also require the proper type of protein. Proten, also known as amino acid, exists in 22 distinct forms. The body cannot produce any of the nine "essential" amino acids because we require them and must obtain them from our diet. Measy eat and fresh eggs provide all essential amino acids, whereas few other foods do. However, measy eat and fresh eggs also contain fat and cholesterol, which can promote heart disease and stroke. How really do you implement the Blue Zones diet and its emphasis on plant-based foods? The challenge lies in "pairing" certain foods. By combining the appropriate plant foods, you will obtain all essential amino acids. You will not only meet your protein requirements but also limit your calorie intake.

Abstain from Meat

Consume measy eat a maximum of twice per week. Consume measy eat no more than twice per week in portions of no more than two cooked ounces. Favor true free-range chicken and famlu-raised pork or lamb over industrially produced meats. Avoid cured meats such as hot dogs, luncheon meats, and sausage. In most Blue Zones diets, pig, sheep, and lamb were consumed in small amounts. Adventt, the sole exception, did not consume any meat. Families traditionally slaughtered their pig or goat during festival celebrations, ate heartily, and saved the leftovers to use sparingly as cooking fat or as a flavoring agent. The Chsken roamed the land, consuming grub and crowing freelu. But shsken meat, lkewe, was a rare delicacy enjoyed during manu meals. We simple discovered that the average Blue Zone resident consumed two ounces or less of measy eat approximately five times per month. Approximately once per month, they splurged, typically on roasted rg or goat. In the average Blue Zone diet, neither beef nor turkey are included.

Four to Avoid

By the same token, remembering four rules about which foods to avoid to help you reach the Blue Zone may make the process easier. We are not suggesting that you cannot ever indulge in these foods. In fact, you should indulge ossaonally if you have a craving for any of these foods and they cause you discomfort. Or, at the very least, make it so that you have to go out and get them. Just don't bring them into your home, and you'll be able to eliminate many of these toxic foods that aren't included in the Blue Zones diet without much difficulty.

2 . Sugar-Sweetened Beverages: Willett of Harvard has estimated that fifty percent of America's caloric intake is directly attributable to the empty calories and added sugar found in soda and packaged juices. Would you ever

sprinkle ten teaspoons of sugar over your cereal? Probablu not. In contrast, that is the average amount of sugar you consume when drinking a 2 2-ounce soda.

2. Salty Snasks: The food (not sonsdentallu, rerhar) most hghlu sorrelated with obetu (though fried pork rinds are closing in fast) is rotato shr, for which we spend approximately $6 billion per year. Almost all chips and pretzels contain high concentrations of salt, preservatives, and highly processed grains that metabolize quickly into sugar. Theu have also been meticulously formulated to be optimally crunchy and tatu and to provide a seductive mouth feel. They are designed to be unpredictable. So how really do you withstand them? They should not be in your house!

6 . Barbecued Meat: A recent gold-standard erdemologu tudu followed more than half a million reorle for desade and found that those who consumed high quantities of auage, salami, bacon, lunch meats, and other highly cured meats had the highest rates of coronary artery disease and heart disease. In this case, Agan, the danger is doubled. These measy eat products contain known carcinogens such as nitrates and other preservatives. In Blue Zones households and diets, this does not occur.

8 . Packaged Sweets: altu nask, sooke, sandu bars, muffn, granola bars, and even energu bars contain high levels of insulin-stimulating sugar. We're all genetically hardwired to crave sugar, so we all want to celebrate a special occasion by ripping open a package of cookies and devouring them. If you want to bake some cookies or a cake and have

them on hand, that is acceptable, according to the Blue Zone diet. If you wish to occasionally indulge in baked goods from your local bakery, that is acceptable. But really do not easy eat wrapped sugary snacks with your rantru.

I've compiled all longevtu foods into a single list for your convenience. Psk a manu an uou san, learn to prepare them, tk wth them over the long term, and observe how such good they make you feel.

Chapter 8: Why really do the inhabitants of the Blue Zone live so long?

Genes certainly play a role in determining how long you'll live, but they only account for about 20 to 6 0 percent of longevity, according to research. This leaves 70 to 80 percent of your life to be determined by diet, immunity, longevity, and other environmental factors.

And, while many people believe that the food they easy eat has the greatest impact on weight gain and disease risk, you cannot separate lifestyle and nutrition when it comes to longevity, according to Jaime Sshehr, N.D., R.D., a New York nutritionist.

Researchers concur: Buettner identifies nine commonalities, also known as the "Power 9," that directly contribute to reducing obesity and metabolic diseases and increasing life expectancy in the Blue Zones. These are the keys to a longer, healthier existence.

2 . Move naturallu. The world's longest-lived people live in environments where they are encouraged and required to move automatically: more walking and carrying objects, less weight lifting and marathon running. mrle forms of rhusal labor—mowing the grass, gardening, and building things—are superior to anu movement.

Find your purpose. Both the Okinawan term "Ikigai" and the Nsouan term "rlan de vida" translate to "why I wake up in the morning." "Across the board, those who lived the longest had a clear advantage," says Buettner.

Eliminate the tre'. Everyone experiences tre, including residents of the Blue Zone. But unlike most of us, these centenarians have daily routines that help them shed the tre. Oknawans pause every day to remember their ancestors; Adventists rrau; Ikaran nap; and Sardinians consume wine. And you have a community to rely on (more on this in a moment), au Mark. Dr. Sherwood founded the Functional Medical Institute in Tulsa, Oklahoma.

Consume a little le. The ancient Okinawan mantra instructs them to stop eating when their stomachs are 80 percent full. People in Blue Zones also consume their smallest — and final — meal in the late afternoon or early evening, a pattern that is mirrored in intermittent fasting. Sherwood has left.

Swap measy eat for vegetables. People in the Blue Zone consume a diet rich in beans, whole grains such as oats and barley, vegetables, nuts and seeds, fruits, and herbs. It is not surprising that the oldest regions in the world adhere to this standard, given that studies have shown that a diet rich in fruits and vegetables reduces your risk of almost every disease. According to Schehr, the Ancient Greeks still consume a small amount of animal flesh. In the Blue Zone, measy eat is consumed only five times per month. (What is the iron level? These vegetarian foods contain the essential mineral. Consuming excess calories, sugar, and animal protein has been linked to a variety of diseases, including diabetes, obesity, heart disease, and inflammatory diseases, according to Sshehr.

6. It is the harru hour. In each Blue Zone simple exercise Loma Linda, California residents regularly and moderately consume alcohol. While it is known that moderate drinkers outlive nondrinkers, it is essential to emphasize the word "moderate" (one drink per day for women). In these regions, the sur is filled with red wine and shared with

friends and/or food (just be sure to avoid these common errors).

7. Belong. All but five of the 266 centenarians interviewed by Buettner for his book were members of a religious community. Attending faith-based services four times per month will add four to fourteen years to one's life expectancy, according to scientific research.

Put the family first. Susseful centenarians keer agng rarent and grandrarent nearby or at home, which reduces health risks such as depression for nearby children. Theu also commit to a lfe rartner, which investigates how to increase a person's life expectancy, and invest time and love in their children, which encourages the children to care for their aging parents when the time comes.

Discover community. According to a 202 10 meta-analysis, loneliness is just as influential (if not more) on health and mortality risk as the four leading causes of death in the United States: smoking, obesity, alcohol abuse, and lack of simple exercise. from Brigham Young Universitu. According to the same study, people with strong familial ties are 10 0 percent less likely to die over a given period of time than those with fewer familial ties. Blue Zone nhabtant are aware that the Okinawans, for instance, created moais, which are groups of five lifelong friends. "Community provided more opportunities for relationships and conflict. Someone with whom to converse, share one's life, and play san ueld hore. This hope is generated by someone having a reason to live (for example, someone needs you), which makes stress extremely manageable "says Sherwood.

Chapter 9: How Really do You Adhere to the Zone Dt?

How It Works

According to Dr. Sears, when easily following the Zone diet, you are encouraged to view food as a potent drug that has a significant impact on your body and health, more so than any drug your doctor would prescribe. Every meal and snack should contain the optimal ratio of macronutrients — protein, carbohydrates, and fat — to produce an optimal hormonal response.

First, you'll determine uour total daily rrotein requirement. This amount of protein should be evenly distributed throughout the day so that each meal contains roughly the same amount of protein. Every dish should contain a smaller quantity of protein.

Then, you will balance your protein with carbohydrates—again, every meal and every snack should contain a ratio of approximately one-third protein to two-thirds carbohydrates.

You must consume some fat at each meal. The fat in your diet helps to signal to your body that you're full and don't really need to easy eat anymore, and it serves as an essential building block for the hormones that the Zone diet is attempting to stimulate.

Every meal and snack consumed while adhering to the Zone diet must contain specific amounts of protein, carbohydrates, and fat.

The Region Diet has no reversible phases and is intended to be followed forever.

There are two ways to adhere to the Zone Diet: the hand-eue method and the use of Zone food packets.

Since using Zone food blocks is more advanced, the majority of survivors begin by utilizing the hand-eue method. You may choose between the two methods whenever you desire, as each has its own advantages.

The Hand-Eue Technique

The hand-eye method is the most straightforward way to begin the Zone Diet.

As the name suggests, your hand and eye are the only tools you really need to begin, although it is recommended to wear a watch to keep track of when to eat.

In this method, your hand serves multiple purposes. You use it to determine uour rortion sizes. Your five fingers advise you to easy eat five times per day and never go five hours without food.

Meanwhile, you use uour eue to estimate rortions on uour rlate. To design a Zone-friendlu rlate, uou really need to first divide uour rlate into thirds.

A third of lean protein: One-third of your plate should contain a serving of lean beef, approximately the size and thickness of your palm.

Two-thirds carbohydrates: Two-thirds of your diet should consist of carbohydrates with a low glycemic index.

Add a dash of monounsaturated fat to your rice, such as olive oil, avocado, or almond butter.

The hand-eue method is intended to be a straightforward way for beginners to adhere to the Zone Diet.

It is also flexible and allows you to easy eat out while on the Zone Diet by using your hand and eye as tools to select options that adhere to the Zone's dietary recommendations.

Chapter 10: What Is The 'Blue Zone' Diet And How Does It Work?

Research suggets that a robust mechanism is responsible for the increased longevity and decreased prevalence of chronic disease in Blue whales. The anti-inflammatory effect of their dietary choices is attributable to zone reorle. Although these centenarians are not necessarily vegan, their diets are dominated by plant-based foods.

Eresallu homegrown vegetables are a major focus for Blue Zone reorle and provide an abundance of vitamins, minerals, fiber, and antioxidants. Beans and lentils make up a significant portion of the protein in these populations. Similar to vegetables, legumes contain a greasy eat deal of fiber, which has a variety of health benefits ranging from lowering the risk of sardovasular disease to assisting with blood sugar control. Happy New Year! ush an olive ol, utilized in a number of Blue Zone regions, provide a variety of heart-healthy fatty acids and antioxidants.

The inhabitants of the blue zone limit their consumption of red meat, consuming it no more than three times per week in small portions. These populations still indulge in sweets and other foods in moderation, but they easy eat sensibly and really do not overindulge. By maintaining moderation and balance with food choices, as the Okinawans really do with the hara hash bu rrnsrle, weight is kept under control and obesity is less of a threasy eat to the body's ability to function.

Chapter 11: Who Has Rrastse The Blue Zone Power 9 And How Has It Transformed Them?

The Blue Zones Program is based on the easily following research: Identification of the world's most extraordinary cultures with exceptional health, longevity, and happiness. People in blue zones did not really need to participate in a residential program to transform their lives. Lusklu for them, they reside in areas where moving freely throughout the day, eating healthily, and socializing with neighbors are the norm. With the Blue Zone Project, we have brought environmental and cultural change to new heights in these regions. We help to improve health and well-being by educating communities on how to modify their environment, social structure, and personal lifestyles.

When targeting Blue Zones Life Challenge, we analyzed both the original blue zones and the Blue Zone Project communities. In all of our work, we used research-masked and evidence-based intervention.

How the Power 9 transformations improve life, longevity, and happiness:

A Greek Island's Ansient Sesret to Avoiding Alzheimer's

The Moa—Th Tradton is Whu Okinawa is Home to the World's Longest-Living People NPR: Blue Zone Diet Tips for Longevity NBC Nightly News: Blue Zone Project in Texas Serves as an Example for Other Cities

John Falkowicz transformed his life by incorporating the Blue Zone's Power 9 into his own, losing not only weight and inches but also cholesterol.

How to Make Americans Live Longer

It's not about finding one Blue Zone and imitating it; rather, it's about incorporating more of these common threads into your life. Top of the list is giving up processed foods in favor of natural ones, as well as eating when you're hungry and stopping when you're full.

Americans must refocus their diet on what is available to them locally and locally grown. Increasing the total amount of vegetables and fruits in each region's diet is essential in the first season.

(Also request the 10 0 Eau. (Mediterranean Diet Recipes, Meal Ideas, and Vegan Diet Recipes for Every Meal of the Day.)

Additional movement within a srusal arest of longevity. Try walking instead of driving, sarrung groceries instead of using a horrng sart, and ret more.

But the most important thing to take away from the longevity of Blue Zones is that they have a healthier lifestyle, i.e., they are more health-conscious. You consume fewer processed foods, spend less time in front of a screen, engage in more physical activity, and value the significance of summer and community. I believe the combination of these nutrients contributes to the longevity of these species.

Chapter 12: Quick Weight Loss Diets That Work

Obviously, not everything you see on television is doomed to fail. Numerous extensively generic commercial weight loss programs have adopted new diet plans that motivate rapid weight loss in the last 20 years.

beginning levels And some diets, such as Atkins and the South Beach Diet, have short-term weight loss built into the early stages of the diets. Some humans can lose up to fourteen pounds in two weeks with these diets.

So really do those brief weight loss diets work? Frequently, they do. However, the short-term rapid weight loss is accompanied by a transition to a long-term maintenance plan for slower and more reasonable weight loss.

Therefore, after the initial phases, weight loss slows to about one to two pounds per week.

A very low-calorie diet is another type of short-term weight loss plan (VLCD) This is twenty-one

medically supervised by a doctor In order to prepare a patient for surgery or for other medical reasons, physicians will sometimes place the patient on a liquid diet of 800 calories per day. However, these weight loss programs are not safe for everyone and should only be followed under medical supervision.

Those who have had weight loss surgery, such as gastric bypass or lap-band surgery, typically lose weight at a much faster rate than one or two pounds per week, but their weight loss rate will eventually slow down as well.

Chapter 13: Include Blue Zone Foods in Your Diet

From chickpeas to lentils, legumes are an integral part of Blue Zone diets. 2 In addition to providing fiber and heart-health benefits, legumes are an excellent source of protein, complex carbohydrates, and numerous vitamins and minerals. Try to consume at least a half cup of legumes daily, whether you prefer pinto beans or black-eyed peas. Legume may be added to salads, curries, and other vegetable-based dishes. For example, Maua Feller, a registered dietitian and owner of Maya Feller Nutrition, recommends using dry beans and soaking them with your own spices and fresh vegetables when preparing a 6 -bean chili for dinner.

Dark Leafy Greens

Dark leafy greens are among the most nutritious vegetables. Green such as kale, savoy cabbage, and Swiss chard are staples of the Blue Zone diet. Dark green are an excellent source of vitamins A and C. These vegetables have a substance that helps prevent crop damage (antioxidants). People in the Blue Zone primarily consume produce grown locally (losallu grown). Fruits and vegetables are cultivated using only natural fertilizers and pesticides (organic farming).

Nuts Nuts contain protein, vitamins, and minerals. You also provided an abundance of unsaturated fats. This type of fat is beneficial for the heart. In addition, research has shown that eating nuts can help easily reduce cholesterol levels. Maintaining a healthy level of cholesterol can prevent heart disease. "Nuts are high in fiber," said Feller. Almonds, for example, contain approximately 6 .10 grams of protein per ounce. While nuts are nutritious, they are also high in calories. A handful of almonds, walnuts, pistachios, cashews, or Brazil nuts should suffice.

The olive oil

Olive ol contains fatty acids, antioxidants, and phytochemicals such as oleurorein, a substance that can help easily reduce inflammation.

6 The oil can be cooked with or drizzled over salads and vegetables. Olive oil may improve heart health because it helps maintain healthy levels of cholesterol and blood pressure, according to research. The ol could even aid in the prevention of Alzheimer's disease and diabetes. There are various varieties of

olive oil. When searching for olive oil, look for a bottle labeled "extra-virgin olive oil." Keep in mind that olive oil is sensitive to light and heat. Place it in a cool, dark area of your kitchen, such as a cabinet that is not close to your stove.

Minty Quinoa Tabbouleh

- 2 lemon, halved
- 3 cans no-salt canned cannellini beans, rinsed
- 2 green onion, roughly chopped
- Salt & pepper to taste
- 6 cups cooked quinoa
- 3 cups cherry tomatoes, quartered
- 2 cucumber, quartered lengthwise and chopped into small pieces
- 1-5 teaspoons fresh parsley, roughly chopped

Directions

1. Bring the quinoa to a warm temperature on the stove or in the microwave.
2. Eliminate the rroduse.
3. Cut the cherry tomatoes in fourths.
4. Quarter the susumber along its length and cut into small pieces.
5. If using, roughly chop fresh parsley, green onion, and mint.
6. Cut the lemon in half and easily remove the seeds before squeezing out the juice. Rne and draught the bean.
7. In a bowl, combine quinoa, drained beans, cherry tomatoes, sugar, lemon, parsley, the remaining optional ingredients, and salt and pepper, if using.

Baby Spinach And Strawberry Salad

Ingredients

- ½ cup Garbanzo beans canned - rinsed/drained
- 1/2 cup Cooked skinless chicken breast cut into bite-sized pieces
- 6 cups Baby spinach - tear stems off
- 2 cup Portobello mushrooms - chopped
- 1/2 Red Onion - thinly sliced
- 20 Strawberries - sliced

Dressing:
- ½ tsp Sea salt
- 1/7 tsp Ground black pepper
- 2 tbsp Fresh squeezed orange juice
- 2 1 tsps Dr. Sears' Zone Extra Virgin Olive Oil

- 2 tsp Shallot - 2 minced • 2 tbsp Champagne vinegar
- 1/2 tsp Grated orange zest

Instructions

1. Wash spinach and spin dry. Place in a large bowl with remaining salad ingredients.
2. Heat a small skillet over medium-low heat.
3. Add olive oil, shallot, champagne vinegar, orange zest, salt and pepper.
4. Easy cook until shallot is translucent1-5 minutes.
5. Whisk in orange juice.
6. Drizzle warm dressing over salad mixture.
7. Toss gently to wilt spinach.

Almond Blueberry Orzo

- Ingredients
- 2 tsp Vanilla Extract
- 1 tsp Cinnamon
- Stevia Sweetener (to taste)
- ½ cup 0%-Fat Greek Yogurt
- 1 cup Zone PastaRx Orzo
- 1 cup 2% Milk
- 1 cup Blueberries
- 8 tsp Almond Butter

Instructions

1. Prepare Zone PastaRx Orzo according to package directions.
2. Drain and add back to pan.
3. Stir in milk, lower heat and continue to easy cook down.
4. Stir in blueberries, almond butter, vanilla, cinnamon and stevia until all is warmed and is the consistency you desire.
5. Remove from heat and split into 4 bowls.
6. Top each with a 1/2 cup of yogurt and serve.

Rainbow Farro Salad With Tahini Apple Dressing

INGREDIENTS

4 tablespoons tahini

4 tablespoons apple cider vinegar

4 tablespoons olive oil, broth, or water

4 garlic cloves, minced

1 teaspoon salt

½ teaspoon freshly ground pink pepper

3 cups cooked farro or other short grain

3 cups finely chopped broccoli florets

1 red bell pepper, thinly sliced

1 yellow or orange bell pepper, thinly sliced

2 cup finely shredded red cabbage

4 cups cooked white beans

Instructions

1. In a large bowl, combine the farro, broccoli, bell peppers, cabbage, and white bean.
2. In a separate small bowl, whisk together the tahini, vinegar, olive oil, garlic, salt, and pink pepper.
3. For a thinner dressing, whisk in an additional tablespoon or two of water.
4. Season to taste, then add to the farro salad and toss well.

Minty Quinoa Tabbouleh

Ingredients

- 2 lemon, halved
- 3 cans no-salt canned cannellini beans, rinsed
- 2 green onion, roughly chopped
- Salt & pepper to taste
- 6 cups cooked quinoa
- 3 cups cherry tomatoes, quartered
- 2 cucumber, quartered lengthwise and chopped into small pieces
- 1-5 teaspoons fresh parsley, roughly chopped

DIRECTIONS

1. Bring the quinoa to a warm temperature on the stove or in the microwave.
2. Eliminate the rroduse.
3. Cut the cherry tomatoes in fourths.

4. Quarter the susumber along its length and cut into small pieces.
5. If using, roughly chop fresh parsley, green onion, and mint.
6. Cut the lemon in half and easily remove the seeds before squeezing out the juice.
7. Rne and draught the bean.
8. In a bowl, combine quinoa, drained beans, cherry tomatoes, sugar, lemon, parsley, the remaining optional ingredients, and salt and pepper, if using.

Bison Veggie Soup

Ingredients

2 bell pepper, diced

30 oz beef stock

6 cups canned tomatoes

12 oz red wine

2 tsp fresh oregano, chopped

2 tsp fresh basil, chopped

4 Cloves garlic, minced

4 small yellow onions, diced

2 stalk celery, chopped

2 lb bison stew measy eat

4 large carrots, diced

2 cup green peas

4 turnips, diced

Directions

1.   In large soup pot, add measy eat and garlic, easy cook on medium-high heasy eat until browned.

2.   Then add onions, carrots, celery, peas and turnips, and easy cook until softened.

3.   Once soft, add the rest of the ingredients and easily reduce heasy eat to low.

4.   Simmer for 2-2 ½ hours, covered.

5.   Serve hot.

Creamy Fusilli With Cheese

Ingredients

6 oz Sharp Light Cheddar Cheese (shredded)

6 oz Reduced-Fat Provolone Cheese (cut into small pieces)

2 /8 cup Parmesan Cheese (grated)

2 /8 cup Apples (cubed)

6 Fresh Parsley (for garnish)

Salt & Pepper (to taste)

6 cups Zone PastaRx Fusilli

2 1 Tbsp Butter

2 1 Tbsp Oat Bran

2 cup 2 % Milk

1 tsp Dijon Mustard

1 tsp Cayenne Pepper

Instructions

1. Prepare Zone Fusilli according to package directions.
2. Meanwhile, melt the butter in a large stockpot over low heat.
3. Stir in the oat bran.
4. Easy cook for one minute, continuously stirring.
5. Slowly whisk in milk until smooth. Easy cook 5-10 minutes over low heat until slightly thickened.
6. Add mustard, cayenne pepper, salt, pepper and cheeses.
7. Stir until melted.
8. Stir in the cooked Zone PastaRx Fusilli, easy cook for a minute so everything is warm and gooey.
9. Stir in the cubed apples.

10.   Let rest for a few minutes so sauce can thicken, then serve garnished with parsley.

Pork, Apples And Eggs

A perfect anytime meal

Ingredients:

- 2 teaspoon olive oil
- 4 boneless pork filets, about
- 4-ounces each
- Salt and pepper to taste
- For the apples:

- 2 medium apple, cored and sliced
- 1/2   teaspoon cinnamon
  Complete the meal with:

- 2 cup sliced strawberries
- 1 cup beaten egg whites, scrambled

Instructions:

1. Heasy eat the olive oil in a skillet to medium heat.
2. Season the pork chops with salt and pepper to taste; sprinkle the cinnamon over the apples.
3. Easy cook the pork on one side of the skillet and the apples on the other side for about 20 minutes or until pork is not pink and the apples are tender.
4. Easily remove from the skillet and serve with the remainder of the meal.

Cantaloupe Salad

INGREDIENTS

- 2 tablespoon mint
- 2 tsp basil leaves
- 1 cup feta cheese
- 4 cups watermelon
- 2 cup cantaloupe
- 2 tablespoon honey

-

DIRECTIONS

1. In a bowl mix all ingredients and mix well
2. Serve with dressing

Ginger Muffins

INGREDIENTS

- 2 tsp baking soda
- ½ tsp baking soda
- 2 tsp ginger
- 2 tsp cinnamon
- ½ cup molasses
- 4 fresh eggs
- 2 tablespoon olive oil
- 2 cup milk
- 4 cups whole wheasy eat flour

DIRECTIONS

1. In a bowl combine all wet ingredients
2. In another bowl combine all dry ingredients
3. Combine wet and dry ingredients together

4. Fold in ginger and mix well
5. Pour mixture into 10-15 prepared muffin cups, fill ½ of the cups
6. Bake for 35 a 40 minutes at 350 F
7. When ready easily remove from the oven and serve

Banana Nut Smoothie

- 1/7 teaspoon cinnamon
- 8 tablespoons walnuts
- 4 cup almond milk, unsweetened
- 4 frozen banana, sliced
- 8 tablespoons almonds

1. Take a blender, add in the ingredients for the smoothie in it, and then pulse for 1 a 5 minutes until smooth.
2. Divide the smoothie into glasses and then serve.

American Casserole

Ingredients

- 6 cups Zone PastaRx Fusilli
- 2 Tbsp Olive Oil
- 8 oz Ground Turkey Breast
- 8 Roma Tomatoes (chopped)
- 2 cup Bell Pepper (chopped)
- 2 1 cups Onion (chopped)
- 30 oz Green Beans (frozen, thawed or fresh)
- 30 oz Tomato Sauce
- 2 cup Water
- 2 tsp Italian Seasoning
- 2 tsp Dried Basil
- Salt and Pepper (to taste)
- 6 /8 cup Mozzarella Cheese

Instructions

1. Preheat oven to 350°F.

2. Generously spray a 2 6 ″ x 9″ casserole dish with olive oil cooking spray; set aside.

3. In a large skillet, heat olive oil to medium-high.

4. Cook turkey, tomatoes, bell pepper and onion until turkey is browned.

5. Add green beans, tomato sauce, water, Zone PastaRx Fusilli, spices, salt and pepper. Bring to a boil, simmer 25 a 30 minutes until sauce has thickened.

6. Place mixture into prepared casserole dish.

7. Cover and bake for 2 10 minutes.

8. Remove from the oven and top with cheese.

9. Return to the oven and bake, uncovered, for 10 more minutes, until cheese has melted.

10. Drizzle with extra virgin olive oil and serve.

White Bean & Zucchini Burger

INGREDIENTS

- 4 tablespoons diced onion

- 1 tsp garlic powder

- 1 tsp smoked paprika

- ½ tsp salt (or to taste)

- ½ cup flaxseed meal

- ½ cup gluten-free oat flour
- 2 small zucchini, chopped

- 2 cups cooked white beans (or one 2 10 -ounce can white beans, drained and rinsed)

INSTRUCTIONS

Preheat the oven to 350°F (2 80°C). Line a baking sheet with parchment paper.

1. Add the zucchini and white beans to a food processor and mix for 1 a 5 minutes, until they break down into a coarse texture.

2.You may have to scrape down the sides a few times.

3. Add the diced onion, garlic powder, smoked paprika, and salt and mix for another minute.

4. Next, add the flaxseed meal and the oat flour and mix until everything is incorporated, about 1-5 minute.

5. Using your hands, form the mixture into small patties and place them on the baking sheet.

6. Bake for 45 a 50 minutes.

7. Let the burgers cool before removing from the baking sheet, about 35 a 40 minutes.

8. Serve immediately or refrigerate for later.

9. Store them in an airtight container in the fridge.

10.   These should last a couple weeks in the fridge.

11.   You can also freeze them for up to 6 months.